NO SUGAR DIET FOR BEGINNERS

An Ultimate Guide To Eliminate Sugar

JOSEPH
LIVINGSTONE

Table of Contents

Introduction

Greetings from the realm of the sugar-free diet! As more people become aware of the negative effects that excessive sugar consumption can have on their health and wellbeing, this dietary strategy has been gaining favor. A no-sugar diet may be the best option for you if you want to gain control over your eating patterns, boost your energy, and enhance your general health.

Since some naturally occurring sugars in whole foods are necessary for a balanced diet, the no-sugar diet does not call for eliminating all sugars. The focus should be on reducing intake of sources of refined and processed sugar and eliminating added sugars.

You'll gain knowledge about how to spot hidden sugars in foods, how to interpret the various names for sugar on ingredient labels, and how to satisfy your sweet need with healthier options as you travel along this path. We will help you develop a meal plan that includes complete foods that are high in nutrients while containing the fewest amount of sugars possible.

While beginning a no-sugar diet may first seem difficult, keep in mind that gradual changes and tiny steps can result in big gains in your health and way of life. Your mood, level of energy, and even your taste preferences will improve over time.

Chapter 1

Introducing No sugar Diet

-Why Choose a No Sugar Diet?

There are several advantages to choosing a no-sugar diet for your health and general wellbeing. Here are some persuasive arguments in favor of a sugar-free diet:

• Weight management: Sugar additions to our diet increase calorie intake without supplying necessary nutrients. A no-sugar diet can assist with weight maintenance and even encourage weight loss by eliminating these worthless calories.

• Improved Blood Sugar Control: People with diabetes or insulin resistance may experience spikes and falls in blood sugar levels as a result of excessive sugar consumption. You can regulate blood sugar levels and increase insulin sensitivity by consuming less sugar.

● Reduced Risk of Chronic Diseases: Type 2 diabetes, heart disease, and some malignancies have all been related to higher risks when it comes to sugar consumption. Adopting a sugar-free diet could reduce these risks and improve long-term health.

● Increased Energy: Although refined sugars can give you a brief energy boost, they frequently cause a crash that leaves you feeling drained and lethargic. You can have more consistent and steady energy levels throughout the day by eliminating sweets.

- Better dental health: Cavities and tooth decay are largely caused by sugar. Limiting your sugar intake can assist safeguard your dental health and lower the likelihood of oral health issues.
- Mental Clarity and Focus: According to some research, consuming too much sugar

may affect cognitive performance and cause brain fog. A sugar-free diet may improve concentration and attention.
- Improved Skin Health: High sugar diets have been linked to skin conditions like acne and early aging. Sugar can contribute to skin that is healthier, brighter, and more vibrant.
- Mood Stability: Sugar highs and crashes might have an impact on mood stability. Reducing sugar consumption may result in a more balanced

emotional state and may lessen the symptoms of depression and anxiety.

● Healthy Eating Habits Are Encouraged: A no-sugar diet pushes you to prioritize full, nutrient-dense meals over processed and sugary alternatives. An overall more nutritious and balanced diet may result from this change.

● Contrary to popular opinion, eating more sugar doesn't necessarily make you crave it less. You can stop the pattern of cravings and lessen your desire for extremely sweet foods by progressively cutting sugar out of your diet.

-Benefits of a No Sugar Diet

● Weight control: A no-sugar diet has a good effect on weight control, which is one of its most noteworthy advantages. You can lower overall calorie consumption and encourage weight loss or maintenance by avoiding or greatly reducing added sugars, especially when combined with a balanced

diet and regular exercise.

• Blood Sugar Levels: By cutting back on foods that cause sudden spikes and drops in blood sugar, a no-sugar diet can help keep levels stable. For those who have diabetes or insulin resistance, this is very advantageous.

• Lower Risk of Chronic Diseases: Excessive sugar consumption has been related to an increased risk of several chronic illnesses, including type 2 diabetes, cardiovascular disease, hypertension, and several malignancies. You may lessen your risk of acquiring these health problems by cutting back on your sugar intake.

• Improved Heart Health: Triglyceride and "bad" LDL cholesterol levels have been found to rise in association with high sugar diets, which are risk factors for heart disease. A sugar-free diet can help lower cholesterol and support better heart health.

• Increased Vitality and Energy: Consuming refined sugars might cause lethargy and energy crashes. You can have more constant energy levels and greater vitality throughout the day by avoiding sweets and concentrating on nutrient-dense diets.

• Increased Mental Clarity and Focus: According to certain research, consuming too much sugar may damage cognitive abilities and cause brain fog. You might have better concentration, mental clarity, and cognitive performance if you cut back on sugar.

● Better Dental Health: Cavities and tooth decay are largely caused by sugary foods and drinks. A sugar-free diet can result in stronger teeth, better dental health, and a lower chance of oral health issues.

● Reduced Anxiety and Balanced Mood: Sugar highs and crashes might have an impact on mood stability. Eliminating sugar from your diet can result in more steady blood sugar levels, which may lessen irritation, anxiety, and mood swings.

● Skin Issues: Acne and early aging of the skin have been related to high sugar diets. You might see brighter, healthier, and more beautiful skin by reducing your sugar intake.

• Reduced Sugar Cravings: Too much sugar consumption can set off a cycle of cravings, making it difficult to resist sweets. This cycle can be broken by a sugar-free diet, which will result in less sugar cravings and a

diminished appetite extremely sweet items.

for

• Promotes Healthy Eating Habits: Adopting a sugar-free diet encourages you to prioritize whole, unprocessed foods that are inherently low in sugar and high in vital nutrients. This change may result in a more wholesome and balanced diet.

• Supports Long-Term Health: A no sugar diet will help you live longer, have a stronger immune system, and feel better overall by lowering your intake of added sugars and choosing healthier foods.

-Understanding Different Types of Sugar

Sugars that occur naturally can be found in a variety of entire foods, including fruits, vegetables, dairy products, and grains. They are a fundamental component of these foods and are packed with important elements like vitamins, minerals, fiber, and antioxidants. Although these sugars are still sugars, they are typically seen as better alternatives when used in a balanced diet. Natural sugars can be found, for instance:

● Fructose is an ingredient in various fruits and root vegetables.

- Glucose The main source of energy for the body is glucose, which is found naturally in many carbs.
- Lactose is a natural sugar found in milk and dairy products.
- Sugars and sweeteners that are included in processed or prepared meals and beverages are referred to as "added sugars." These sugars, also known as "empty calories," have little to no nutritional benefit. Multiple health problems might result from consuming too much added sugar. It is crucial to carefully examine food labels because added sugars may be mentioned on ingredient labels under several names. Several popular sweeteners and added sugars include:
- Frequently used in baking and cooking, sucrose (table sugar) is a mixture of glucose and fructose.

- Sweetener High Fructose Corn Syrup (HFCS): This substance is frequently found in baked products, soft drinks, and processed foods.
- Often used as a sweetener and in some processed goods, dextrose is another term for glucose.
- Maltose is a starch-derived sugar that is frequently present in beer and malted beverages.
- Honey: A bees' natural sweetener that, when added to food, is still regarded as sugar.
- A sweetener derived from maple tree sap is called maple syrup.

Chapter 2

Getting Started with Your No Sugar Diet

-Assessing Your Current Sugar Intake

● Keep a Food Journal: To begin, log your meals in great detail for at least a week. Include meals, snacks, and beverages in the list of everything you consume. Make sure to record the serving sizes and quantities.

● Recognize Sugary Foods and Beverages: Look over your food journal and note any foods or beverages that have added sugars. Sugary snacks, sweets, sweetened beverages (such as soda, energy drinks, sweetened teas, etc.), and processed meals with added sugars (such as cereals, sauces, dressings, etc.) may be included in this list.

- Read Food Labels: Acquire the ability to read food labels and look for added sugars in the ingredients list. Be aware that added sugars can go by a variety of names, including sucrose, high fructose corn syrup, dextrose, maltose, and others. Pay close attention to the amount of sugar in each dish.
- Calculate Your Daily Sugar Intake: Using the information from your food journal and the nutritional facts on food labels, total up all the grams of added sugar you consume daily. You may see your current daily sugar intake from this.
- Recognize Hidden Sugars: Be aware of sugars that may be present in foods that may appear to be healthy, such as yogurt, granola bars, and flavored

oatmeal. These goods may have significant sugar additions.

● Examine Beverages: Consider your beverage selections carefully because they may be substantial sources of extra sugars. High sugar intake can be caused by sugary sodas, sweetened coffee drinks, fruit juices, and energy drinks.

● Comparing your calculated daily sugar intake to the advised amounts will help you understand the recommended sugar intake. The American Heart Association recommends limiting daily added sugar consumption to no more than 25 grams (or 6 teaspoons) for women and 36 grams (or 9 teaspoons) for men.

● Establish Realistic Goals: Based on your evaluation, establish reasonable objectives for lowering your sugar intake. You could begin by gradually reducing your intake of sugary snacks and switching to water or unsweetened beverages in place of sweetened ones.

● Plan Balanced Meals: Pay attention to putting together a variety of full, nutrient-dense foods in your meals while limiting the intake of items that are high in added sugars. Increase your intake of fruits, veggies, lean proteins, and whole grains.

● Seek Support: If you're having trouble determining how much sugar you're consuming or changing your diet, think about getting help from a qualified dietitian or nutritionist. They may offer you individualized advice and assist you in making a plan that is suited to your requirements and tastes.

- Setting Realistic Goals

Consider making modest changes to your diet rather than trying to completely cut out added sugars overnight. You may start by, for instance, avoiding sugar-sweetened beverages or cutting back on the sugar in your coffee or tea. A modification made gradually has a higher chance of sticking and developing into a habit.

● Choose Particular

Set definite, objectives for Instead of a general objective like "eat less sugar," specify steps you can take, such as "limit dessert to once a week" or "substitute fresh fruit for sugary snacks."

● Be Aware of Hidden Sugars: Be aware of any sugars that may be present in packaged foods and condiments. Make it a point to check food labels

Actions: defined yourself and steer clear of items with a lot of sugar. Your decision-making will improve as a result of this routine.

• Set Daily or Weekly limitations: Set daily or weekly limitations for the consumption of added sugar. You may, for instance, try to adhere to the American Heart Association's advice and limit your intake to no more than 25 grams (or about 6 teaspoons) for women and 36 grams (or about 9 teaspoons) for men per day.

• Create balanced meals with a range of nutrient-rich foods by concentrating on planning them. Making it a point to include more nutritious grains, lean meats, fruits, and veggies in your meals will inevitably lead to less room for sweets.

● Permit Occasional Treats: Completely depriving yourself of all sweets may not be a long-term solution. Instead, reward yourself with the odd treat for maintaining your sugar-free diet plan. Modesty is important.

● Keep a log of your sugar intake and the steps you take to reach your objectives. This can be done by keeping a meal journal, using a smartphone app, or just taking notes. You may maintain accountability and motivation through tracking.

● Seek Support: Discuss your no-sugar-added diet objectives with loved ones, close friends, or online communities. Having a support network can offer inspiration, drive, and practical advice.

● Take Care of Yourself: Recognize that switching to a sugar-free diet may provide some difficulties. Don't be too hard on yourself if you make mistakes or have setbacks every now and then. Instead of concentrating on perfection, try to make progress, and treat any failures as teaching moments.

● Acknowledge and celebrate your accomplishments, no matter how minor they may seem. Every effort made to reduce added sugar consumption is a step in the right direction toward greater health.

- Creating a Meal Plan

A good method to remain on track with your sugar-free diet and make sure you are choosing balanced and healthful foods is to make a meal plan. You can design a meal plan that supports your no-sugar lifestyle using the step-by-step instructions provided below:

● Set Your Daily Caloric Needs: Determine how many calories you need each day depending on your age, gender, amount of exercise, and weight objectives. The portion proportions and overall meal planning will be based on this.

● Include a Variety of Food Groups: To make sure you're getting all the necessary nutrients, try to include a variety of food groups in your meals. Include fresh produce, whole grains, lean proteins, healthy fats, dairy products (if preferred), and fruits and vegetables.

● Focus on entire Foods: Whenever feasible, choose entire, unprocessed foods. These foods have better nutritional value and naturally have less added sugar.

- Plan for Three Main Meals and Snacks: Create a daily food schedule that includes three well-balanced main meals (breakfast, lunch, and dinner) and wholesome snacks. This will help to keep energy levels steady and stop excessive hunger.
- Decide on Low-Sugar Breakfasts: Start your day with low-sugar breakfast selections. Choose whole-grain cereals, oats prepared the night before, sugar-free smoothies, or eggs topped with vegetables.
- Create lunch and dinner options without sugar: Focus on eating meals at lunch and dinner that are high in veggies, lean proteins, and healthy fats. Include grilled proteins, salads, stir-fries, and vegetable-based soups.

- Plan wholesome, satiating snacks devoid of added sugars as an alternative to unhealthy snacking. Fresh fruit, almonds, plain Greek yogurt, hummus-dipped carrot sticks, and homemade energy snacks made with dates are a few ideas.
- Make water your main beverage throughout the day to stay hydrated. Avoid fruit juices and other sugar-filled beverages. To add taste, you can infuse water with herbs or fresh fruits.
- Prepare and batch-cook: Take into account preparing and cooking a few meals and snacks ahead of time. During hectic days, this will save time and lessen the temptation to go for bad options.
- Be Creative with Your Recipes: Experiment with new dishes that are naturally low in sugar or utilize natural

sweeteners. Online and in cookbooks, there are a ton of delectable sugar-free recipes to choose from.

• Plan for Eating Out: If you frequently dine out, look up places that provide low- or no-sugar menus. By looking at the menu online in advance, you can choose healthier options.

• Be adaptable: Keep in mind that a meal plan is a suggestion, not a set of rigid rules. Be versatile and flexible, particularly when unforeseen circumstances or cravings emerge. As necessary, alter your meal plan while keeping in mind your no-sugar objectives.

Chapter 3

Identifying Hidden Sugars

-Reading Food Labels

In order to determine whether packaged foods include added sugars, reading product labels is crucial while following a no-sugar diet. To read food labels correctly, remember the following advice:

● First, glance at the ingredients list to see whether there are any added sugars. The quantity of an ingredient is indicated in the product by its position on the ingredient list, which is sorted by weight and is presented in descending order. Look for words that imply sugar, such as sucrose, high fructose corn syrup, dextrose, maltose, or any word that ends in "-ose."

• Be on the lookout for Hidden Sugars: Even items that don't taste sweet can have added sugars. Beware of sugar lurking in unexpected places like condiments, pasta sauces, and salad dressings.

• Recognize Sugar Terminology: To make sugar less visible, food makers may use multiple names for it. Learn the different names and sweeteners, such as honey, agave nectar, maple syrup, and molasses, that are used to describe sugar.

• Look at the nutrition information panel: On the Nutrition Facts panel, have a look at the "Total Sugars" section. Both the product's added and natural sugars are included in this figure. Remember that added sugars are those that are added during manufacturing, whereas natural sugars come from sources like fruits and dairy.

● Serving Sizes: Pay attention to the serving size that is specified on the label. Until you discover that it is based on a smaller serving size than you usually eat, the amount of sugar can seem modest.

● Watch Out for Sugar-Free Claims: Be wary of items that claim to be "sugar-free" or "no sugar added." Despite the fact that these items may not have added sugar, they may nevertheless contain natural sugars or sugar substitutes.

● Choosing between comparable products requires comparison of their sugar contents. Select the product using natural sweeteners or the one with the least amount of added sugar.

• Select entire Foods: Emphasizing entire, unprocessed foods is the greatest approach to stay away from added sugars. In general, whole grains, lean meats, fruits, and vegetables have little to no added sugars.

• Avoid Low-Fat Products at All Costs: Products that are low in fat or fat-free frequently make up for the loss of flavor by increasing their sugar content. To be sure you're not drinking too much added sugar, read the labels.

• Avoid highly processed foods because they are more likely to include added sugars, especially if they have a long list of ingredients. Reduce the intake of these goods you consume.

-Sneaky Names for Sugar in Ingredient Lists

Sucrose is a type of table sugar that contains both glucose and fructose.

● High Fructose maize Syrup (HFCS) is a sweetener typically found in processed foods and beverages. It is manufactured from maize starch.

● Another name for glucose is dextrose, which is frequently used as a sweetener and in some processed foods.

● Fructose is a naturally occurring sugar that can be found in honey and fruits, but it is also used to sweeten food products.

● Maltose is a starch-derived sugar that is frequently present in beer and malted beverages.

- Glucose syrup is a sweetener produced by hydrolyzing starch that is used in many processed goods.
- High fructose corn syrup can be substituted with brown rice syrup, a sweetener derived from brown rice.
- A sweetener made from agave plants, agave nectar is frequently found in natural and healthy food products.
- When used in processed foods, maple syrup—a natural sweetener derived from the sap of maple trees—still counts as additional sugar.
- Honey: A naturally occurring sweetener made by bees, however when added to food, it's seen as extra sugar.
- A sweetener created by hydrolyzing sucrose into its glucose and fructose components is known as invert sugar.

- High fructose corn syrup-like sweetener derived from corn starch is known as corn syrup.
- A sweetener prepared from malted barley, barley malt syrup is frequently used in a variety of dishes and drinks.
- Beet sugar is a type of added sugar that is made from sugar beets.
- Powdered sugar, also referred to as confectioner's sugar, is made by combining finely pulverized sugar with cornstarch.
- Turbinado Sugar: A sugar that has been partially refined and still contains some molasses.
- Unrefined whole cane sugar known as panela is frequently used in several cuisines.
- High fructose corn syrup can be replaced with rice bran syrup, a sweetener made from rice bran.

To make better educated decisions about the foods you eat, keep an eye out for these sly aliases for sugar when reading ingredient labels. When feasible, choose whole, unprocessed foods to lower your overall intake of added sugars and boost the nutritious value of your diet.

Chapter 4

Foods to Avoid on a No Sugar Diet

-High-Sugar Fruits and Vegetables
While most fruits and vegetables are healthful and full of vital nutrients, some varieties have higher concentrations of natural sugars than others. It's crucial to be aware of the fruits and vegetables you eat if you're on a no-sugar diet or trying to reduce your sugar intake. Here are some examples of fruits and vegetables with a lot of sugar:
Sugar-Rich Fruits:
● Grapes Cherries
● Watermelon
● Pineapple Figs
● Lychees

- Mangoes
- Tangerines
- Pomegranates
- Bananas:

These fruits continue to be wholesome and offer essential vitamins, minerals, and dietary fiber. But if you're worried about how much sugar they contain, think about consuming them in moderation and concentrating more on lower-sugar alternatives.

Fruits with less sugar:

- Strawberries, blueberries, raspberries, etc.
- Avocado
- Kiwi
- Cantaloupe Papaya Peaches
- Plums
- Apricots Oranges
- Apples

These fruits are excellent options for anyone looking to cut back on sugar because they have less natural sugar than other fruits.

Vegetables High in Sugar:
● Beets
● Carrots
● Winter Squash (like butternut squash) Peas
● Corn
These veggies provide important nutrients, much like fruits, but have a higher natural sugar content. When ingesting them, pay attention to the portion proportions.
Less-Sugar Produce:
● Arugula or spinach
● Broccoli
● Cauliflower
● Peppers, bell

- Cucumbers
- Tomatoes
- Zucchini
- Eggplant
- Brussels Sprouts
- Asparagus

These veggies are ideal options for a no-sugar diet because they have reduced natural sugar content.

-Processed Foods and Sugary Snacks
Added sugars in processed foods:

- Breakfast Cereals: There are a lot of breakfast cereals with a lot of added sugar, especially those targeted toward kids.
- Sweetened Yogurt: Yogurts with flavors and fruit on the bottom frequently have sugars added. Choose plain Greek yogurt and sweeten with

fresh fruit or a thin drizzle of natural honey.

• Sauces in a can or bottle: Many sauces, including ketchup, barbecue sauce, and teriyaki sauce, have sugar added for flavor.

• Salad dressings: Some commercial salad dressings may be highly sweetened. Make your own dressing at home or look for ones without extra sugar.

• Packaged foods: Added sugars are frequently present in processed foods including cookies, cakes, muffins, and granola bars.

• Drinks with Added Sugars: The main sources of added sugars include soda, energy drinks, sweetened teas, and fruit juices. Instead, choose unsweetened beverages, herbal teas, or water.

● Coffee creamers with flavors: Sugar is frequently added to flavor creamers. Use unsweetened substitutes like coconut or almond milk.

● Packets of instant oatmeal: Instant oatmeal that comes in a package may be practical, but it frequently has extra sugar. Pick plain oats and combine them with your favorite natural sweeteners and toppings.

Sugary Foods:

● Candy and chocolate: Snacks with limited nutritional value and a high added sugar content include sweets, chocolate bars, and gummies.

● Donuts and pastries: These sweets are frequently laden with sugar and bad fats.

● Frozen desserts and ice cream: Many frozen desserts and ice cream have a lot of added sugar.

- Sugary Cereal Bars: Many cereal bars are actually very heavy in sugar, while being advertised as a healthier snack.
- Flavored Popcorn: Some flavors of flavored popcorn, particularly the sweet ones, may contain additional sugars.
- Check the labels when purchasing dried fruits because some varieties have sugars added.
- Pre-packaged trail mixes frequently include sweetened dried fruits and candies, which raises the sugar intake. Sweetened nuts and trail mixes.

It's better to minimize or stay away from these processed meals and sugary snacks when trying to follow a no-sugar diet. Pick entire, unprocessed foods instead, such as lean proteins, fruits, vegetables, whole grains, nuts, and seeds. You may manage your sugar intake and make healthier decisions by preparing meals and snacks at home with natural sweeteners like honey, maple syrup, or fruits. In order to support your general health and wellbeing, keep in mind to carefully read food labels and prioritize whole foods.

-Sugary Beverages and Alternatives
drinks that are sweet:
Regular Coke is among the worst offenders because it has a lot of added sugars.
● Fruit juices: Even 100% fruit juices can have considerable natural sugar content, and many commercial kinds also contain added sugars.
● Teas that have been sweetened: Sweet teas that are sold in cans and

bottles frequently have a lot of extra sugar added to them.

● Energy drinks: These alcoholic beverages are frequently laced with sugar and caffeine.

● Waters with Flavors: Sugar and artificial sweeteners may be added to flavored water drinks.

● Sports beverages: For casual physical activity, sports drinks are frequently unnecessary
and may contain extra sugars.

Drinks That Are Better For You:

Water is the healthiest and most hydrating option. Fresh fruit or herbs can be used to naturally flavor water without the addition of sugar.

● Teas made from herbs: Teas made from herbs, especially those without additional sweeteners, are typically reviving and devoid of added sugars.

- Choose unsweetened sparkling water for a bubbly and delightful alternative.
- Black or green tea are both excellent options because they are unsweetened and include antioxidants as well as a small amount of caffeine.
- Homemade Fruit-Infused Water: To make homemade fruit-infused water, combine normal water with fresh fruit slices such as lemon, lime, berries, or cucumber.
- Unsweetened iced tea can be made at home by brewing your own unsweetened tea and, if preferred, sprinkling on some lemon or honey.
- Coffee with Minimal Additives: A healthy alternative to regular coffee is black coffee, coffee with a tiny amount of unsweetened milk,

or coffee with natural sweeteners like cinnamon.

Chapter 5

Meal Prep and Recipes

-No Sugar Breakfast Ideas
Setting a healthy tone for the rest of the day with a no-sugar-added breakfast in the morning is a great idea. Here are some tempting and healthy no-sugar breakfast suggestions:

• Greek Yogurt Parfait: For a rich and filling breakfast, layer unsweetened Greek yogurt with fresh fruit, almond slices, and a dash of cinnamon.

• Eggs are whisked and then poured over bell peppers, mushrooms, spinach, and other sautéed vegetables to make a vegetable omelet. Avocado slices can be put on top for further richness.

• Chia Seed Pudding: Blend chia seeds with unsweetened coconut milk or almond milk and refrigerate overnight. Add some fresh fruit on top and, if you'd like, a drizzle of honey or maple syrup as a natural sweetener.

• Prepare oatmeal with unsweetened almond milk or water. Oatmeal with nuts and seeds. Add fresh fruit, such as sliced bananas or berries, chopped almonds, chia seeds, and flaxseeds over the top.

• Smoothie Bowl: Blend spinach, frozen berries, unsweetened almond milk, and a scoop of protein powder (free of added sugars) to make a filling and tasty smoothie bowl. Add extra berries, hemp seeds, and unsweetened coconut flakes on top.

- Avocado Toast: Spread mashed avocado over whole-wheat toast and top with sliced tomatoes, salt, pepper, and olive oil.
- Scrambled eggs, sautéed vegetables, and a dollop of plain Greek yogurt for extra richness may all be combined to a whole-grain tortilla to make a vegetarian breakfast burrito.
- Wrapped in a whole-wheat tortilla, this breakfast sandwich of smoked salmon, cream cheese, cucumber slices, and arugula is quick to prepare and high in protein.
- Smoothie with unsweetened shredded coconut, chia seeds, and a dash of vanilla extract is made using coconut milk and other tropical ingredients.
- Chopped nuts, fresh fruit, and a drizzle of agave nectar or date puree

are added to cooked quinoa in a bowl along with water or unsweetened almond milk.

-Sugar-Free Lunch and Dinner Recipes
Quinoa salad and lemon herb chicken on the grill:
Marinate chicken breasts in a mixture of olive oil, garlic, thyme, rosemary, and lemon juice. Cook completely on the grill.
Over a bed of quinoa salad that has been combined with diced cucumbers, cherry tomatoes, red onions, and fresh parsley, serve the grilled chicken. Dress with olive oil, lemon juice, Dijon mustard, salt, and pepper-based lemon vinaigrette.

Salmon Baked with Roasted Veggies:

Put salmon filets on a baking pan. Add your chosen herbs and salt & pepper to taste. Salmon should be baked until flaky.

Olive oil, garlic, and herbs are used to roast a range of vegetables, such as broccoli, cauliflower, and bell peppers, until they are soft. Serve the roasted veggies with the fish.

Pesto-topped zucchini noodles with grilled shrimp You may make zucchini noodles by spiralizing them. They should be cooked till soft in a pan with olive oil.

Blend fresh basil, garlic, pine nuts, olive oil, and Parmesan cheese to create a pesto without sugar. Add grilled shrimp to the pesto-coated zucchini noodles.

Lettuce wraps with turkey and avocado:

In a skillet, cook lean ground turkey with onions, garlic, and your preferred seasonings.

Place the cooked turkey mixture, avocado slices, sliced tomatoes, and a dollop of Greek yogurt for creaminess on top of the large lettuce leaves. Wraps can be made by rolling up lettuce leaves.

Fried rice with cauliflower and tofu:

Pulse cauliflower florets In a food processor until they look like rice. Cook the cauliflower rice in tamari sauce (gluten-free soy sauce) while adding diced tofu, mixed vegetables, and other seasonings.

Bell Pepper Stuffed:

Remove the tops and seeds from

bell peppers. The peppers should be parboiled for a few minutes to slightly soften them.

Make a filling by sautéing diced tomatoes, cooked quinoa, onions, garlic, and lean ground turkey or beef. Bake the peppers until they are soft after stuffing them with the mixture.

Stir-Fried Lentils and Veggies:

Cook lentils as directed on the packaging. Stir-fry a variety of colorful veggies with garlic and ginger in a separate skillet, including broccoli, snap peas, carrots, and bell peppers.

Serve over brown rice or cauliflower rice after combining the cooked lentils with the stir-fried vegetables and seasoning with low-sodium soy sauce.

fettuccine squash with tomato-basil sauce:

Spaghetti squash should be roasted until soft. With a fork, remove the strands.

Garlic, onions, and chopped tomatoes are sautéed in olive oil with fresh basil, salt, and pepper to make a sugar-free tomato basil sauce. Spaghetti squash should be topped with sauce.

- Healthy Snack Options

Healthy snacks can support your no-sugar diet while also being satiating and nourishing, giving you enduring energy throughout the day. Here are a few delectable sugar-free snack choices:

• Fresh Fruit: Sample a variety of fruits that are still in season, such as apples, berries, oranges, grapes, or sliced melon. Fruits have a built-in sweetness and are a great source of vitamins, fiber, and antioxidants.

• Cut up celery sticks, carrot sticks, cucumber slices, bell pepper strips, or other vegetables for a crisp and nourishing snack, and serve them with a dish of hummus.

• Nuts and Seeds: Pumpkin or sunflower seeds, coupled with a handful of unsalted nuts like almonds, walnuts, or cashews, provide a filling and protein-rich snack.

• Greek yogurt: Choose plain, unsweetened Greek yogurt and flavor it with fresh berries, a dash of cinnamon, or (in moderation) a drizzle of honey.

• Whole-grain rice cakes spread with natural peanut or almond butter provide a tasty and satisfying snack.

● Fill rice paper with avocado, avocado slices, cooked shrimp, or cooked tofu for rice paper rolls. For a quick and healthy snack, dunk them in a no sugar-added dipping sauce.

● Homemade Trail Mix: To make your own trail mix, combine a variety of unsweetened nuts, seeds, and dried fruits, such as unsweetened coconut, goji berries, or dried apricots.

● Popcorn: For a flavorful and filling snack, air-pop plain popcorn and season with nutritional yeast, garlic powder, or your preferred herbs.

● Cucumber Avocado Bites: Place cherry tomatoes, mashed avocado, and a dash of salt and pepper on top of cucumber slices.

● Dark Chocolate: Opt for dark chocolate with at least a 70% cocoa content to avoid the sugar that milk chocolate usually contains. Take a nibble for a tasty pleasure.

- Roasted Chickpeas: For a salty, protein-rich snack, toss cooked chickpeas with olive

oil and your preferred seasonings.

- Cottage Cheese and Berries: For a creamy, high-protein snack, combine cottage cheese and fresh berries.

- Vegetable Chips: To make your own vegetable chips, slice vegetables such as sweet potatoes, zucchini, or beets very thinly and bake them in the oven until they are crisp.

- Chia Seed Pudding: To make chia seed pudding, use unsweetened almond milk. For sweetness, top it with fresh fruit.

- Sliced cheese and whole-grain crackers: This tasty snack combines protein and fiber-rich sliced cheese with whole-grain crackers.

Chapter 6

Overcoming Sugar Cravings

-Understanding the Causes of Cravings Strong wants for particular foods or flavors are known as cravings, and they can be difficult to control. The emergence of cravings is influenced by a variety of physiological, psychological, and environmental factors. Here are a few typical reasons for cravings:

● Nutritional Deficiencies: Cravings may indicate that your body is deficient in a certain nutrient. For instance, eating chocolate can be a clue that you need more magnesium, whereas craving salty treats might be a sign that you need more sodium.

• Rapid fluctuations in blood sugar can make people crave sweet or high-carb foods in an effort to normalize their blood sugar levels.

• Emotional triggers include stress, anxiety, boredom, and other feelings that can result in emotional eating and desires for comfort foods that are frequently heavy in sugar, fat, and salt.

• Habitual Eating: Consuming a particular food repeatedly might lead to habitual desires because your brain links a particular flavor or texture to reward or pleasure.

• Social and environmental cues: Cravings can be sparked by outside influences like ads, social circumstances, or even witnessing someone else consume a certain item.

• Dopamine Response: Some foods, especially those high in sugar and fat, can stimulate the reward system in the brain, causing the release of dopamine, a neurotransmitter linked to motivation and pleasure. Due to this, a cycle of desire and reward-seeking behavior could develop.

• Cravings can be learnt by positive associations made throughout childhood or other life experiences, which is referred to as a learned behavior.

• Hormonal Changes: Food desires may change as a result of hormonal changes during menstruation, pregnancy, or menopause.

● Sleep Deprivation: Sleep deprivation can alter hunger hormones and heighten desires for foods high in calories.

● Food Addiction: According to some study, some very appetizing and processed meals may cause the brain to react in a way that is similar to addiction, resulting in cravings and a lack of control over food intake.

You can effectively manage and minimize cravings if you are aware of their underlying causes. Here are some methods for overcoming cravings:

● Keep Hydrated: Sometimes, hunger or desires might be confused for thirst. To stay hydrated, routinely consume water.

● Eat Balanced Meals: To help regulate blood sugar levels and lessen cravings, prioritize balanced meals that include a variety of proteins, healthy fats, and complex carbohydrates.

● Eat slowly to enjoy your meals and pay heed to your body's signals of hunger and fullness.

● Identify healthy coping mechanisms for stress and emotions, such as exercise, meditation, or hobbies.

● Get Enough Sleep: To support general health and curb cravings, strive for ample and quality sleep.

● When cravings arise, choose healthier substitutes that will satisfy your palate without throwing off your sugar-free diet.

● To avoid feelings of deprivation from creeping in and also to minimize potential eating episodes, do well to practice moderation by allowing yourself occasional treats.

● Plan ahead and keep wholesome snacks on hand to avoid impulsive decisions when cravings strike.

-Strategies to Cope with Cravings
Dealing with cravings can be difficult, particularly if you're attempting to stick to a sugar-free diet or make healthier decisions. You can, however, control and get rid of cravings with a few techniques and practice. Here are some practical methods for overcoming cravings:

● Distract Yourself: When a hunger strikes, try to divert your attention by getting involved in anything else. To divert your attention from the urge, go for a stroll, read a book, make a phone call, engage in a pastime, or start a new one.

• Recognize Your Triggers: Recognize what makes you crave certain foods. Stress, feelings, particular locations, or even certain hours of the day, could be the cause. You
can start working on developing healthy ways to react to triggers once you've identified them.

• Become more attentive of your thoughts and sensations regarding desires by practicing mindfulness. Without passing judgment, acknowledge the craving and allow it to pass without giving in. You can learn to pay closer attention to your body's messages through meditation or mindful breathing.

• Remind yourself that you can indulge in the meal or treat later when a craving strikes. Delaying pleasure allows you to reconsider if you actually need or want the object.

• Select Healthier Options: If you're in the want for something sweet, choose a piece of fresh fruit or a modest serving of a dessert that is naturally sweetened. Choose nuts and seeds or veggie sticks with hummus if you're in the mood for something crunchy.

• Keep Hydrated: Thirst can occasionally be confused with hunger or cravings. After consuming a glass of water, wait a while to observe whether the urge goes away.

• Create a Meal Plan: Making a meal plan with wholesome, filling meals might help lessen cravings. To feel full and nourished, make sure your meals contain a variety of proteins, good fats, and complex carbohydrates.

● Get Enough Sleep: Not getting enough sleep can lead to increased desires, particularly for items high in sugar and calories. Make sleeping well a priority to boost your general wellbeing.

● Don't Keep Tempting Foods Around: If you are aware that specific foods cause intense cravings, try not to keep them close at hand. Out of sight, out of memory is a cycle that can be broken.

● Exercise Moderation: It's important to give yourself periodic indulgences in moderation even while you're trying to cut back on your sugar intake.

● Seek Support: Discuss your no-sugar diet adventure with friends, family, or a support group. It might be motivating to have someone with whom to discuss your difficulties and achievements.

- **Forgive Yourself:** If you do occasionally give in to a craving, accept responsibility for it and move on. Refrain from feeling guilty and concentrate on future healthier decisions.

Chapter 7

The Role of Exercise in a No Sugar Lifestyle

-Exercise and Blood Sugar Regulation

• Increased Insulin Sensitivity: Consistent exercise raises the body's insulin sensitivity. A hormone called insulin aids in the movement of glucose from the bloodstream into cells, where it can be used as fuel. Improved sensitivity makes cells more receptive to insulin and reduces the amount of insulin needed to transport glucose into the cells, improving blood sugar control.

• Greater Uptake of Glucose: During exercise, active muscles use more glucose. This enhanced muscle cell absorption of glucose lowers blood sugar levels.

- Lessened Insulin Resistance: Insulin resistance is a condition in which cells react less favorably to insulin, which makes it challenging for glucose to enter the cells. Regular exercise can assist to lessen insulin resistance, improving control.

blood sugar of Glycogen: depletes the muscles' glycogen stores. Withdrawing glucose from the plasma to restore glycogen after exercise can help

- Utilization Exercise

reduce blood sugar levels.

- Better Weight Management: Regular exercise can help you maintain your weight or lose weight, which is especially good for people with type 2 diabetes or prediabetes. A healthy weight is maintained, which helps with blood sugar regulation.

• Post-Exercise Effect: The advantages of exercise for controlling blood sugar levels can persist after the workout. According to several studies, exercising can improve insulin sensitivity for several hours after exercise.

• Exercise can aid in reducing stress, which is important because stress hormones can cause blood sugar levels to rise.

It's crucial to remember that the effect of exercise on blood sugar levels can change based on a number of variables, including the kind, degree, and length of exercise, one's level of fitness, and dietary preferences. In order to create a customized fitness program that is appropriate for their requirements and medical situation, people with diabetes or those at risk of developing the disease should collaborate with their healthcare team, which should include doctors and trained diabetes educators

-Incorporating Physical Activity into Your Routine
You can lead a healthier and more active lifestyle by including physical activity in your daily routine. Numerous advantages of regular exercise include improved cardiovascular health, better mood, stress reduction, weight control, and blood sugar regulation, among others. Here are some suggestions to assist you in including regular physical activity in your daily routine:
● Create Achievable Exercise Goals Based on Your Current Fitness Level

and Schedule, Create Achievable Exercise Goals is the first step. As you get more accustomed to regular exercise, gradually up the intensity and length of your workouts.

● Pick Activities You Enjoy: Look for physical activities you actually enjoy. If you enjoy what you're doing, you're more likely to stick with it over the long haul whether you're dancing, swimming,
hiking, biking, practicing yoga, or playing a sport.

● Schedule Exercise Time: Include time for exercise in your daily or weekly schedule to treat it as a priority. Make physical activity a non-negotiable component of your day by blocking out particular periods for it on your schedule.

- Begin Slowly: To avoid injury and gradually increase your fitness level, start with low-impact exercises or shorter sessions if you are new to exercise or haven't been active in a while.
- Be Consistent: Developing a habit of exercising requires consistency. Try to include some form of exercise in your routine most days of the week, even if it is only for a short while.
- Be Active Throughout the Day: Even if you are unable to schedule specific training time, look for opportunities to be active throughout the day. Use the stairs rather than the elevator, travel by foot or bicycle to local locations, or engage in quick bouts of activity when you have a break.
- Mix It Up: Change workouts to enable things to go smooth and fresh.

To keep yourself from getting bored and to push your body, try a variety of workouts.

● Find a Workout Partner: Working out with a buddy can increase motivation and accountability while also making sessions more fun.

● Pay Attention to Your Body: During and after exercise, pay close attention to how your body feels. It's natural to experience some stiffness in the muscles, but if you feel pain or discomfort, take a day off from exercising or adjust your routines as necessary.

● Celebrate Your Progress: No matter how tiny, acknowledge and honor your successes. You may stay motivated and dedicated to your exercise goals by monitoring your progress.

- Make it a Family Event: If at all feasible, get the whole family moving. Family game nights, bike trips, and walks may all be enjoyable ways to stay active as a unit.

Chapter 8

Long-Term Health Benefits

Numerous long-term health advantages can result from frequent physical activity and leading an active lifestyle. These advantages affect your whole well-being in a positive way and go beyond just the physical. The following are a few long-term health advantages of frequent exercise:

Cardiovascular Health: Consistent exercise fortifies the heart and enhances cardiovascular health. It can lower blood pressure, enhance blood circulation, and lessen the risk of heart disease.

Weight management: By burning calories and gaining lean muscle mass, exercise aids in weight management. When used in conjunction with a healthy diet, it can help people lose weight and prevent weight gain.

Blood Sugar Control: Regular exercise increases insulin sensitivity and lowers blood sugar levels in people with diabetes and those at risk of developing the disease.

Bone Health: Weight-bearing activities such as jogging, walking, and resistance training help improve bone density and lower the risk of osteoporosis.
Exercise has numerous positive effects on mental health. It can lessen the

signs of anxiety and sadness, lift your spirits, and sharpen your mind.

Sleep Quality: Regular exercise encourages improved sleep habits and raises the standard of sleep.

Immune Function: Moderate exercise can strengthen your immune system and lower your risk of contracting certain infections and diseases.
Joint Health: Movement and exercise on a regular basis can assist to increase joint flexibility and lower the risk of disorders related to the joints.

Energy Levels: Exercise increases energy and decreases symptoms of weariness.

Longevity: In older persons, regular exercise is linked to both a longer lifespan and higher quality of life.

Cognitive Health: Exercise may help lower the risk of cognitive decline and neurodegenerative illnesses and is thought to have a good effect on brain health.

Stress Reduction: Exercise helps lower stress levels and foster relaxation and overall well being.

Social Engagement: Taking part in team sports or group exercise courses can offer chances for social engagement and community involvement, which improves general well-being. Self-Confidence: Reaching physical milestones and reaping the rewards of consistent exercise can increase one's sense of self-worth and self-confidence.

Remember that these long-term health advantages do not materialize instantly. experience these benefits, physical activity must be practiced consistently and with a commitment. It's also important to select pursuits you can stick with over the long term. Finding activities that you enjoy will make it simpler to permanently incorporate them into your routine, To whether you choose to exercise by walking, dancing, cycling, swimming, or any other activity.

www.ingramcontent.com/pod-product-compliance
Lightning Source LLC
Chambersburg PA
CBHW070822280726
48660CB00017B/2387